Nurturing Babies Naturally

A Mother's Guide to Naturopathic Baby Care

Vidya shankar

Table Of Contents

Chapter 1: Introduction to Naturopathic Baby Care

Understanding Naturopathic Medicine

In this subchapter, we will delve into the fascinating world of naturopathic medicine and how it can benefit your baby's health and well-being. Naturopathic medicine is a holistic approach to healthcare that focuses on the body's innate ability to heal itself. By addressing the root causes of illness and promoting overall wellness, naturopathic medicine offers a gentle and natural way to care for your baby.

One of the fundamental principles of naturopathic medicine is the belief in the healing power of nature. Naturopathic doctors (NDs) recognize that the human body has an inherent ability to heal and restore balance. Through the use of natural remedies, such as herbs, supplements, and homeopathy, naturopathic medicine supports the body's healing process while minimizing the use of pharmaceutical drugs and invasive procedures.

Naturopathic medicine also emphasizes the importance of prevention and education. By focusing on lifestyle factors, such as nutrition, sleep, and stress management, naturopathic doctors empower parents to make informed choices that promote their baby's optimal health. They work closely with mothers to develop personalized care plans that address the unique needs of each child, taking into consideration their age, developmental stage, and individual health concerns.

Unlike conventional medicine, which often treats symptoms in isolation, naturopathic medicine takes a comprehensive approach to healthcare. NDs consider the interconnectedness of the body and how various systems, such as the digestive, immune, and nervous systems, influence one another. By addressing the underlying imbalances that contribute to illness, naturopathic medicine aims to restore harmony and promote long-term health.

Furthermore, naturopathic medicine embraces a patient-centered approach. NDs strive to create a nurturing and supportive environment where mothers feel heard, respected, and actively involved in their baby's care. They take the time to listen to your concerns, ask detailed questions about your baby's health history, and conduct thorough physical examinations to gain a holistic understanding of your child's well-being.

In conclusion, understanding naturopathic medicine is crucial for mothers seeking a natural and holistic approach to baby care. By harnessing the healing power of nature, promoting prevention, and considering the whole person, naturopathic medicine offers a gentle yet effective way to nurture your baby's health naturally. This subchapter will provide you with a comprehensive overview of the principles and benefits of naturopathic medicine, empowering you to make informed choices for your little one's well-being.

Benefits of Naturopathic Baby Care

Naturopathic baby care is an approach that focuses on the natural and holistic well-being of your little one. By incorporating natural remedies, healthy lifestyle choices, and gentle therapies, it aims to support your baby's overall health and development. In this subchapter, we will explore the numerous benefits of naturopathic baby care and how it can positively impact your child's life.

1. Support for the Immune System: Naturopathic baby care emphasizes boosting your baby's immune system naturally. Through natural remedies, such as herbal supplements and homeopathic remedies, you can strengthen your baby's defenses against common illnesses like colds, flu, and digestive issues.

2. Gentle and Safe Treatments: Naturopathic baby care focuses on using gentle and safe treatments that are free from harmful chemicals and additives. This approach ensures that your baby's delicate system is not exposed to unnecessary toxins, reducing the risk of adverse reactions or side effects.

3. Promotes Healthy Growth and Development: Naturopathic baby care encourages healthy growth and development through proper nutrition and lifestyle choices. It emphasizes the importance of breastfeeding, introducing nutrient-rich solid foods, and creating a nurturing environment that supports your baby's physical, emotional, and cognitive development.

4. Preventative Approach: One of the key benefits of naturopathic baby care is its preventative approach. By addressing potential health issues before they arise, you can minimize the chances of your baby experiencing common ailments. Through regular check-ups, nutritional guidance, and natural remedies, naturopathic care helps prevent health problems and promotes optimal well-being.

5. Individualized Care: Every baby is unique, and naturopathic baby care recognizes this by providing individualized care tailored to your baby's specific needs. By understanding your baby's constitution, temperament, and health history, naturopathic practitioners can create personalized treatment plans that support your baby's unique journey towards wellness.

6. Empowers Mothers: Naturopathic baby care empowers mothers by providing them with knowledge and tools to care for their babies naturally. This approach encourages active involvement and fosters a deeper understanding of your baby's health needs, allowing you to make informed decisions and ensure the well-being of your little one.

In conclusion, naturopathic baby care offers a wide range of benefits that promote the natural health and well-being of your baby. By embracing this approach, you can support your baby's immune system, promote healthy growth and development, and take a preventative approach to their health. With its individualized care and emphasis on safe and gentle treatments, naturopathic baby care empowers mothers to provide the best possible care for their little ones, nurturing them naturally.

The Role of Mothers in Naturopathic Baby Care

As a mother, your role in providing naturopathic baby care is vital for your child's overall well-being and development. In this subchapter, we will delve into the significant role you play in nurturing your baby naturally and how you can incorporate naturopathic principles into your baby's care routine.

Naturopathic baby care focuses on using natural remedies and approaches to enhance your baby's health and prevent illnesses. It recognizes that babies have unique needs and aims to support their innate healing abilities. As a mother, you are the primary caregiver and have a profound influence on your baby's health. By adopting naturopathic principles, you can promote optimal health for your little one.

One essential aspect of naturopathic baby care is breastfeeding. Breast milk provides the ideal nutrition for your baby, containing essential nutrients and antibodies that boost their immune system. As a mother, your role is to ensure proper latch and positioning, establish a breastfeeding routine, and maintain a healthy diet to produce quality breast milk.

Additionally, you can incorporate naturopathic practices into your baby's daily care routine. This includes using natural and organic products for bathing and skincare, avoiding harsh chemicals and toxins that can harm your baby's delicate skin. You can also incorporate gentle baby massage techniques, which not only promote bonding but also aid in digestion, relaxation, and overall well-being.

Another crucial role you play as a mother is in promoting a healthy environment for your baby. Naturopathic baby care emphasizes creating a toxin-free and nurturing space for your little one. This involves using natural cleaning products, ensuring proper ventilation, and minimizing exposure to harmful substances such as tobacco smoke or synthetic fragrances.

Furthermore, you are responsible for making informed decisions regarding your baby's healthcare. Naturopathic approaches encourage a holistic view of health and seek to address the root cause of any illness or discomfort. As a mother, you can work closely with a naturopathic doctor or healthcare provider to explore alternative treatments, herbal remedies, and dietary adjustments that may benefit your baby's health.

In conclusion, the role of mothers in naturopathic baby care is indispensable. By embracing natural approaches, breastfeeding, incorporating gentle techniques, creating a healthy environment, and making informed healthcare decisions, you can provide your baby with the best start in life. This subchapter aims to empower you with the knowledge and tools necessary to nurture your baby naturally and ensure their overall well-being.

Chapter 2: Preparing for a Naturopathic Baby

Creating a Natural and Safe Environment

In this subchapter, we will explore the importance of creating a natural and safe environment for your baby. As a mother, you want nothing but the best for your little one, and adopting a naturopathic approach to baby care can help you achieve just that.

First and foremost, it is essential to understand the significance of a natural environment for your baby's overall well-being. By embracing natural materials and products, you ensure that your baby is not exposed to harmful chemicals, toxins, or synthetic substances that can negatively impact their health. Opt for organic cotton clothing, bedding, and toys to minimize exposure to pesticides and other harmful substances.

Additionally, consider the air quality in your baby's environment. Indoor air can often be more polluted than outdoor air, so it is crucial to take measures to improve air circulation and quality. Keep the windows open whenever possible to allow fresh air in and use natural air purifiers such as plants to filter out toxins. Avoid using synthetic air fresheners, cleaning products, or other chemical-laden substances that can compromise your baby's respiratory health.

Creating a safe environment goes hand in hand with a natural one. Baby-proofing your home is essential to prevent accidents and injuries. Install safety gates, secure heavy furniture to the walls, cover electrical outlets, and ensure that all hazardous items are out of reach. Use non-toxic cleaning products to maintain cleanliness without exposing your baby to harmful chemicals.

In this subchapter, we will also discuss the importance of natural light and its impact on your baby's sleep patterns, mood, and overall development. Exposing your baby to natural light during the day can help regulate their circadian rhythm, resulting in better sleep quality. Ensure that your baby's sleeping area is not overly exposed to artificial light sources such as screens or bright nightlights, as these can disrupt their sleep patterns.

By creating a natural and safe environment for your baby, you are providing them with the best possible start in life. A naturopathic approach to baby care prioritizes your baby's health and well-being by minimizing exposure to harmful substances and creating a nurturing space for them to grow and thrive.

Remember, as a mother, you have the power to shape your baby's environment and create a foundation for a healthy and happy life. Embrace the naturopathic way of baby care and watch your little one flourish in a natural and safe environment.

Choosing Naturopathic Healthcare Providers

When it comes to the health and well-being of our precious little ones, as mothers, we always want the very best. This is why choosing the right healthcare provider for our babies is of utmost importance. In this subchapter, we will delve into the key factors to consider when selecting a naturopathic healthcare provider for your baby, ensuring that you are making an informed and confident decision.

First and foremost, it is essential to do thorough research. Look for naturopathic doctors who specialize in baby care and have a wealth of experience in this field. Check their credentials, certifications, and educational background to ensure their expertise aligns with your preferences. Reading reviews and testimonials from other mothers who have sought their services can also provide valuable insights.

Another crucial aspect to consider is compatibility. A naturopathic healthcare provider should be someone you feel comfortable discussing your concerns and asking questions. They should have a warm and approachable demeanor, putting both you and your baby at ease during consultations. Trust and open communication are vital for creating a strong bond between the provider, mother, and baby.

Assessing their treatment approach is equally important. Naturopathic medicine focuses on a holistic and natural approach to healthcare, seeking to address the root cause of any ailments rather than merely alleviating symptoms. Ensure that the provider follows this philosophy and incorporates it into their practice. They should be knowledgeable about natural remedies, nutrition, and lifestyle modifications that can support your baby's overall health and well-being.

It is also advisable to consider the location and accessibility of the naturopathic healthcare provider. Having a provider who is conveniently located and easily accessible will save you time and effort, especially during those unexpected moments when your baby requires immediate attention.

Lastly, trust your instincts. As a mother, you possess a unique intuition that often guides you towards what is best for your baby. If you have any reservations or doubts about a particular healthcare provider, it may be worth exploring other options until you find someone with whom you feel completely comfortable and confident.

In conclusion, choosing a naturopathic healthcare provider for your baby requires careful consideration. By conducting thorough research, assessing compatibility, treatment approach, location, and trusting your instincts, you can ensure that you find the perfect healthcare provider who will nurture and support your baby's natural health journey. Remember, you are your baby's advocate, and making an informed choice will set your little one on the path to optimal wellness.

Developing a Support Network

As a mother, one of the most important aspects of caring for your baby is to establish a strong and reliable support network. While the journey of motherhood can be incredibly rewarding, it can also be overwhelming and challenging at times. Having a support system in place can make all the difference in navigating the ups and downs of raising your baby naturally, the naturopathic way.

A support network can consist of various individuals who can provide emotional, practical, and informational support throughout your journey. These individuals can include family members, friends, fellow mothers, and even healthcare professionals who share your beliefs in naturopathic baby care.

Family members, especially grandparents, can be a valuable source of support and wisdom. Their experience and knowledge can offer guidance and reassurance during moments of uncertainty. Friends who are also parents can be an excellent source of empathy and understanding, as they have likely faced similar challenges and can share their own experiences and advice.

Joining a community of fellow mothers who embrace naturopathic baby care can provide a sense of belonging and camaraderie. This community can be found through local support groups, online forums, or even social media platforms. Connecting with like-minded individuals can help alleviate feelings of isolation and provide a safe space to ask questions, seek guidance, and share successes and challenges.

Healthcare professionals who specialize in naturopathic baby care can also play a crucial role in developing your support network. Seek out naturopathic doctors, pediatricians, or lactation consultants who are knowledgeable and supportive of your natural approach. Their expertise can guide you in making informed decisions about your baby's health, wellness, and natural remedies that align with your goals.

In addition to these individuals, it is essential to educate yourself about naturopathic baby care through reliable sources such as books, websites, and reputable organizations. Arm yourself with knowledge about natural remedies, breastfeeding, nutrition, and other aspects of caring for your baby naturally. This knowledge will empower you to make informed decisions and advocate for your baby's well-being.

Remember, developing a support network is not a sign of weakness but rather a testament to your commitment to providing the best possible care for your baby. By surrounding yourself with individuals who understand and support your naturopathic approach, you will find confidence, reassurance, and a sense of community throughout your motherhood journey.

Chapter 3: Naturopathic Nutrition for Babies

Breastfeeding and its Benefits

Breastfeeding is a natural and beautiful way for mothers to nourish and bond with their babies. In this subchapter, we will explore the numerous benefits of breastfeeding for both mother and baby, highlighting how this natural approach aligns with the principles of naturopathic baby care.

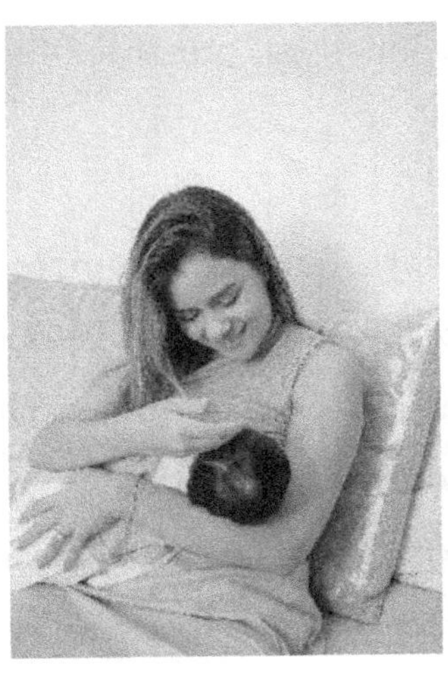

Breast milk is often referred to as "liquid gold" due to its remarkable composition. It contains a perfect blend of essential nutrients, antibodies, and enzymes that are specifically tailored to meet the needs of a growing baby.

Unlike formula milk, breast milk is easily digestible, reducing the risk of digestive issues and allergies. It also provides optimal hydration, preventing constipation and promoting healthy bowel movements.

One of the most significant benefits of breastfeeding is the boost it provides to the baby's immune system. Breast milk is rich in antibodies that help protect against a wide range of infections and diseases. This natural immunity transfer is especially vital during the first six months when a baby's immune system is still developing. Breastfed babies have been shown to have fewer respiratory illnesses, ear infections, and gastrointestinal issues.

For mothers, breastfeeding offers numerous advantages as well. It stimulates the release of oxytocin, a hormone that promotes relaxation and bonding. This intimate connection between mother and baby can enhance emotional well-being and reduce postpartum depression. Additionally, breastfeeding helps mothers lose pregnancy weight more rapidly as it burns calories and contracts the uterus.

From a naturopathic perspective, breastfeeding aligns perfectly with the principles of gentle and natural baby care. It avoids the use of artificial substances found in formula milk, which may contain additives, preservatives, or synthetic nutrients. Breast milk ensures that babies receive the purest and most natural form of nutrition, supporting their overall growth and development.

Breastfeeding also promotes a healthy gut microbiome, which is crucial for a strong immune system and optimal digestion. The beneficial bacteria present in breast milk help populate the baby's gut, establishing a foundation for a robust and balanced microbiota.

In conclusion, breastfeeding is a fundamental aspect of naturopathic baby care, offering a multitude of benefits for both mother and baby. By choosing to breastfeed, mothers can provide their little ones with optimal nutrition, enhanced immunity, and a deeper emotional connection. The unique composition of breast milk, along with its natural and gentle qualities, makes it the perfect choice for nurturing babies naturally.

Introducing Solid Foods Naturally

As a mother, your baby's health and well-being are your top priorities. When it comes to introducing solid foods, the naturopathic way provides a natural, healthy approach that supports your baby's development. In this subchapter, we will explore the benefits of introducing solid foods naturally and provide you with practical tips to navigate this important milestone.

Naturopathic baby care emphasizes the use of whole, unprocessed foods to nourish your baby's growing body. By introducing solid foods naturally, you can ensure that your little one receives all the essential nutrients needed for optimal development. Unlike processed baby foods, which often contain additives and preservatives, natural foods provide a wide range of vitamins, minerals, and antioxidants that support your baby's immune system and overall health.

Before starting solid foods, it is crucial to observe your baby's readiness cues. Look for signs such as sitting up with minimal support, showing interest in food, and the ability to move food from the front of the mouth to the back. These signs indicate that your baby's digestive system is maturing and ready to handle solid foods.

When selecting the first foods for your baby, opt for nutrient-dense options such as mashed avocado, sweet potato, or pureed fruits like bananas or pears. These foods are easy to digest and provide essential vitamins and minerals. Start with a small amount and gradually increase the quantity as your baby develops a taste for solid foods.

To enhance the nutritional value of solid foods, consider introducing homemade bone broths or vegetable purees. Bone broths provide important minerals like calcium and phosphorus, while vegetable purees offer a variety of vitamins and fiber. By making your baby's food at home, you have control over the ingredients and can ensure that only the freshest, organic options are used.

It is essential to introduce one new food at a time and observe any allergic reactions or digestive issues. By doing this, you can identify potential food sensitivities or allergies and make adjustments accordingly. Additionally, be mindful of introducing allergenic foods such as peanuts, dairy, or eggs, and consult with a naturopathic doctor if you have concerns.

Introducing solid foods naturally is a beautiful journey that allows you to nourish your baby's body and lay the foundation for a lifetime of healthy eating habits. By following these naturopathic principles, you can provide your little one with the best start in life, supporting their growth and development every step of the way.

Promoting Healthy Eating Habits

One of the most important aspects of naturopathic baby care is promoting healthy eating habits right from the start. As a mother, you play a crucial role in shaping your baby's diet and setting the foundation for a lifetime of good health. In this subchapter, we will explore the key principles and strategies for nourishing your baby naturally.

Introducing Solid Foods

When it comes to introducing solid foods, it is recommended to follow your baby's cues and introduce them gradually. Start with simple, homemade purees made from organic fruits and vegetables. Avoid processed foods, as they often contain additives and preservatives that can be harmful to your baby's delicate system. By making your own baby food, you have control over the ingredients and can ensure that your little one is getting the best nutrition possible.

Breastfeeding and Formula Feeding

Breastfeeding is the ideal way to nourish your baby, providing essential nutrients and antibodies that boost their immune system. If breastfeeding is not an option, choose a high-quality organic formula that closely mimics breast milk. Avoid formulas that contain artificial ingredients, sugars, or genetically modified organisms (GMOs). It's essential to establish a healthy feeding routine and create a peaceful environment during feeding times to promote bonding and relaxation.

Avoiding Allergenic Foods

Food allergies are becoming increasingly common, and it's important to be mindful of potential allergens when introducing solids. Start with single-ingredient foods, such as pureed fruits or vegetables, and wait a few days before introducing a new food to observe any allergic reactions. Common allergenic foods, such as dairy, wheat, nuts, and shellfish, should be introduced later, around 8-10 months of age, to reduce the risk of allergies.

Creating a Balanced Plate

As your baby grows, it's important to provide a variety of foods to meet their nutritional needs. Aim for a balanced plate that includes a combination of fruits, vegetables, whole grains, and proteins. Incorporate a rainbow of colors to ensure a diverse range of vitamins and minerals. Avoid processed snacks and sugary drinks, as they can contribute to obesity and other health issues later in life.

Establishing Healthy Eating Habits

By setting a positive example and involving your baby in meal preparation, you can establish healthy eating habits from an early age. Encourage self-feeding and offer a wide variety of textures and flavors. Avoid using food as a reward or punishment, as this can lead to emotional eating patterns. Instead, focus on creating a peaceful and enjoyable mealtime experience where your baby can explore and appreciate different foods.

In conclusion, promoting healthy eating habits is a vital part of naturopathic baby care. By following these principles and strategies, you can nourish your baby naturally and set them on a path to a lifetime of good health. Remember, every baby is unique, so be flexible and responsive to their individual needs.

Chapter 4: Natural Remedies for Common Baby Ailments

Understanding the Principles of Natural Remedies

In the modern world, where synthetic medicines and treatments dominate the healthcare industry, more and more mothers are turning to natural remedies for their baby's care. In this subchapter, we will explore the principles behind natural remedies and how they can benefit your baby's well-being.

First and foremost, it is essential to understand that natural remedies aim to support and strengthen the body's own healing mechanisms. Unlike conventional medicine, which often focuses on suppressing symptoms, natural remedies foster a holistic approach to healing, addressing the root cause of the issue rather than just the symptoms. This approach resonates well with the naturopathic philosophy of treating the whole person, considering their physical, mental, and emotional well-being.

One of the fundamental principles of natural remedies is the use of plant-based ingredients. Herbs, essential oils, and other botanicals are often central to naturopathic baby care. These natural substances contain a wide array of beneficial compounds that can support your baby's health in various ways. From soothing chamomile tea for colic to calendula-infused creams for diaper rash, plants provide gentle yet effective solutions.

Another principle to understand is the importance of nourishing and supporting your baby's immune system. Natural remedies focus on providing the body with the necessary tools to fight off illness and maintain optimal health. This can involve using immune-boosting herbs and supplements, ensuring a nutrient-rich diet, and creating a healthy environment free from toxins.

Furthermore, natural remedies prioritize prevention rather than just treatment. By adopting a proactive approach, mothers can reduce the likelihood of their baby falling ill and promote overall well-being. This includes practices such as breastfeeding, implementing a balanced diet, promoting good hygiene, and using natural remedies to support the body's defenses.

It is worth noting that while natural remedies can be incredibly beneficial, it is essential to consult with a qualified naturopathic practitioner or healthcare professional before embarking on any new treatments. They can provide personalized guidance based on your baby's specific needs and health history.

By understanding the principles of natural remedies, mothers can provide their babies with a naturopathic approach to care. This holistic and gentle approach can support their baby's overall health and well-being, ensuring a strong foundation for a lifetime of wellness.

Treating Digestive Issues Naturally

As a mother, there is nothing more distressing than seeing your baby suffer from digestive issues. From colic to constipation, these conditions can be incredibly uncomfortable for your little one, leaving you feeling helpless. However, there are natural remedies and techniques that can effectively address digestive problems in babies, providing relief without the use of harsh medications. In this subchapter, we will explore the naturopathic approach to treating digestive issues in babies, empowering you with the knowledge and tools to nurture your baby naturally.

One of the first steps in addressing digestive issues naturally is to understand the importance of proper nutrition. Breast milk is the ideal food for infants, as it contains all the necessary nutrients and enzymes to promote healthy digestion. If breastfeeding is not an option, opting for organic formula can be a good alternative. Additionally, introducing solid foods gradually and focusing on homemade, nutrient-rich purees can help support your baby's digestive system.

Next, we will delve into the power of probiotics. Probiotics are beneficial bacteria that can restore the natural balance in your baby's gut. They can be found in fermented foods like yogurts and kefir. Adding a small amount of probiotic-rich foods to your baby's diet can improve digestion and alleviate common digestive issues such as gas and bloating.

In this subchapter, we will also explore the benefits of herbal remedies for digestive problems. Gentle herbs like chamomile and fennel can be used to soothe an upset stomach or relieve colic symptoms. We will discuss how to prepare herbal teas or infusions and the proper dosage for your baby's age.

Additionally, we will cover the importance of proper feeding techniques, such as burping your baby after each feeding and avoiding overfeeding, which can contribute to digestive issues. We will provide practical tips on how to create a calm and relaxed feeding environment to enhance digestion.

Finally, we will touch upon the significance of addressing any underlying causes of digestive issues, such as food sensitivities or allergies. We will guide you on how to identify potential triggers and provide suggestions for an elimination diet to identify problematic foods.

By incorporating these natural approaches to treating digestive issues, you can help your baby find relief and promote optimal digestive health. This subchapter aims to empower you as a mother to confidently nurture your baby naturally, providing them with the best possible care for their digestive well-being.

When it comes to herbal teas or infusions for babies, it's important to exercise caution as some herbs may not be suitable for infants. It is generally recommended to avoid giving herbal teas to infants under six months of age. After six months, you can gradually introduce certain herbal teas in small quantities, but it's advisable to consult with your pediatrician before doing so. The dosage and specific herbs can vary based on the baby's age, health, and individual circumstances.

Here are a few herbal teas that are sometimes used for babies and their appropriate dosages:

1. Chamomile Tea: Chamomile tea is known for its calming properties and can be helpful for soothing an upset stomach or aiding sleep. For infants over six months, you can start with a small amount (around 1-2 ounces) of weak chamomile tea, diluted with boiled and cooled water. It's best to start with a very weak brew and gradually increase strength if needed. However, it's important to note that some infants may be allergic to chamomile, so closely monitor for any adverse reactions.

2. Fennel Tea: Fennel tea is often used to alleviate colic symptoms and aid digestion. It's generally safe for infants over six months.

Start with a weak fennel tea infusion by steeping 1 teaspoon of crushed fennel seeds in 8 ounces of boiled and cooled water. Give a small amount (1-2 ounces) to your baby and observe for any adverse effects. However, it's essential to note that fennel tea should not be given to infants with epilepsy or a history of seizures.

3. Peppermint Tea: Peppermint tea can help with digestive issues such as gas and bloating. However, it's best to avoid giving peppermint tea to infants under one year of age due to the potential risk of triggering reflux or reducing milk supply in breastfeeding mothers.

If you decide to introduce peppermint tea after one year, consult with your pediatrician for appropriate dosage and preparation.

4. Rooibos Tea: Rooibos tea is a caffeine-free herbal tea that is generally safe for babies and toddlers. It's rich in antioxidants and has a mild, naturally sweet taste. You can offer small amounts of weak rooibos tea to your baby as a beverage, but avoid adding any sweeteners. Remember, it's crucial to consult with your pediatrician before introducing any herbal tea or infusion to your baby's diet.

They can provide personalized guidance based on your baby's specific needs and any potential allergies or health conditions.

Soothing Skin Conditions with Natural Remedies

As a mother, one of your top priorities is keeping your baby healthy and happy. However, sometimes little ones can experience skin conditions that cause discomfort and worry.

Fortunately, there are natural remedies available to help soothe these issues and provide relief for your precious bundle of joy. In this subchapter of "Nurturing Babies Naturally: A Mother's Guide to Naturopathic Baby Care," we will explore some effective ways to address common skin conditions using the principles of naturopathy.

Skin conditions can vary from mild irritations to more severe rashes, and they can be caused by a variety of factors such as allergies, environmental irritants, or even genetics. Regardless of the cause, using natural remedies can often provide relief without the need for harsh chemicals or medications.

One of the most common skin conditions in babies is diaper rash. To soothe this discomfort, you can try using natural remedies such as coconut oil or calendula cream, which have soothing and healing properties. These gentle ingredients can help reduce inflammation and promote healing without causing any harm to your baby's delicate skin.

Another skin condition that may affect babies is eczema, characterized by dry and itchy patches. A naturopathic approach to managing eczema involves identifying and avoiding potential triggers such as certain foods or environmental factors. Additionally, using natural moisturizers like shea butter or chamomile-infused oils can help keep the skin hydrated and reduce inflammation.

For babies with cradle cap, a common condition characterized by flaky and crusty patches on the scalp, you can try massaging a small amount of olive oil or almond oil onto the affected area. This will help loosen the flakes, making them easier to remove during gentle washing.

Naturopathy focuses on using natural remedies and lifestyle modifications to support overall health and wellness. When addressing common skin conditions in a one-year-old baby, here are some effective ways to consider using the principles of naturopathy:

1. Maintain a Healthy Diet: A balanced and nutrient-rich diet is crucial for healthy skin. Ensure that your baby's diet includes plenty of fruits, vegetables, whole grains, and healthy fats like avocados and nuts. Avoid processed foods, sugary snacks, and foods that may trigger allergies or sensitivities.

2. Hydration: Keep your baby well-hydrated by offering them water frequently. Sufficient hydration helps maintain skin moisture and overall health.

3. Gentle Bathing: Use lukewarm water for bathing and limit the bath time to avoid drying out the skin. Avoid using harsh soaps or cleansers and opt for mild, natural, and fragrance-free products specifically formulated for babies.

4. Moisturize Naturally: After bathing, apply a natural, gentle, and hypoallergenic moisturizer to keep the skin hydrated. Look for ingredients like aloe vera, shea butter, coconut oil, or calendula, which can be soothing and nourishing for the skin.

5. Avoid Irritants: Be mindful of potential irritants that can aggravate skin conditions.This includes harsh chemicals, fragrances, synthetic fabrics, and certain detergents. Opt for natural and hypoallergenic products, use fragrance-free laundry detergents, and dress your baby in soft, breathable clothing made from natural fabrics like cotton.

6. Calendula Oil or Cream: Calendula has soothing and anti-inflammatory properties that can be beneficial for various skin conditions. Apply a small amount of calendula oil or cream to the affected areas as directed by a qualified naturopathic practitioner or pediatrician.

7. Oatmeal Baths: Oatmeal has soothing properties and can help relieve itching and inflammation. You can place a small amount of finely ground oats in a muslin cloth or oatmeal bath product specifically made for babies and add it to the bathwater. Gently rub the cloth over your baby's skin to release the soothing properties.

8. Probiotics: Probiotics, either in the form of a supplement or through foods like yogurt, can support gut health and balance the immune system. A healthy gut can positively impact the skin. Consult with a healthcare professional regarding appropriate probiotic options and dosages for your baby's age. 9.

It's important to note that while natural remedies can be effective, each baby is unique, and what works for one may not work for another. It's always a good idea to consult with a naturopathic doctor or pediatrician to ensure the best course of action for your baby's specific needs.

In this subchapter, we have explored some natural remedies to soothe common skin conditions in babies. By embracing the principles of naturopathy and utilizing these gentle remedies, you can provide relief for your little one without resorting to harsh chemicals or medications. Remember, a happy and healthy baby begins with a mother's nurturing touch and the power of nature's remedies.

Chapter 5: Promoting Natural Sleep and Relaxation

Establishing Healthy Sleep Patterns

Sleep is essential for the overall health and well-being of both babies and their mothers. It is during sleep that the body repairs, restores, and rejuvenates itself. However, many new mothers struggle to establish healthy sleep patterns for their babies. In this subchapter, we will explore the naturopathic approach to nurturing babies' sleep, providing practical tips and strategies to promote restful and rejuvenating sleep for both baby and mother.

First and foremost, it is important to understand that babies have their own unique sleep needs. While some babies may sleep through the night from an early age, others may need more frequent awakenings for feeding or comfort. By recognizing and respecting these individual differences, mothers can better meet their baby's sleep requirements.

Creating a soothing sleep environment is crucial for establishing healthy sleep patterns. Begin by ensuring the baby's sleep space is calm, quiet, and free from distractions. Soft lighting, such as a dim nightlight, can help create a peaceful atmosphere. Additionally, using natural bedding materials and avoiding synthetic fragrances can contribute to a more serene sleep environment.

Establishing a consistent bedtime routine can signal to the baby that it is time to sleep. This routine can include activities such as a warm bath, gentle massage, or a soothing lullaby. By repeating this routine every night, babies will begin to associate these activities with sleep, making the transition to bedtime smoother.

Naturopathic remedies can also play a role in promoting healthy sleep patterns for babies. Gentle, natural remedies like chamomile tea or lavender-infused bathwater can have a calming effect and aid in relaxation. However, it is always important to consult with a qualified naturopathic practitioner or healthcare provider before introducing any new remedies to your baby.

Mothers should also prioritize their own sleep and well-being. Taking care of oneself is crucial for being able to care for a baby effectively. Establishing a support system, whether through a partner, family, or friends, can provide much-needed rest and rejuvenation for mothers.

In conclusion, establishing healthy sleep patterns for babies is essential for their overall well-being. By creating a soothing sleep environment, implementing a consistent bedtime routine, and incorporating naturopathic remedies, mothers can nurture their babies' sleep in a natural and holistic manner. Prioritizing self-care and seeking support is also vital to ensure that both mother and baby are well-rested and thriving.

Creating a Relaxing Bedtime Routine

A good night's sleep is essential for both babies and their mothers. As a mother, you want your little one to sleep peacefully, ensuring their optimal growth and development. In the book "Nurturing Babies Naturally: A Mother's Guide to Naturopathic Baby Care," we explore the naturopathic way of caring for your baby, including the importance of establishing a relaxing bedtime routine.

1. Set a Consistent Bedtime: Babies thrive on routine, so it's essential to establish a consistent bedtime. Choose a time that works best for your family and stick to it every night. This helps regulate your baby's internal clock, making it easier for them to fall asleep and wake up at the desired times.

2. Create a Calming Environment: Transform your baby's sleep area into a calming sanctuary. Dim the lights, play soft, soothing music, and maintain a comfortable temperature. Consider using a white noise machine or a gentle fan to create a consistent background sound that can drown out any sudden noises that may disrupt your baby's sleep.

3. Establish a Relaxing Bedtime Ritual: A consistent routine signals to your baby that it's time to wind down and prepare for sleep. Start with a warm bath using natural, chemical-free baby products. This can help relax your baby's muscles and soothe their senses. Follow the bath with a gentle baby massage using natural oils, such as lavender or chamomile, known for their calming properties.

4. Engage in Quiet Activities: After the bath, engage in quiet, low-stimulation activities such as cuddling, singing lullabies, or reading a bedtime story. Choose books with soothing tones and gentle illustrations to create a peaceful atmosphere. Avoid stimulating activities or toys that may excite your baby and make it harder for them to settle down.

5. Breastfeed or Bottle-feed: If your baby is still young and requires a feeding before bed, try to create a peaceful feeding environment. Dim the lights and keep the atmosphere calm and quiet. Avoid stimulating your baby with excessive talking or playfulness. After the feeding, gently burp your baby and hold them upright for a few minutes to prevent discomfort.

Remember, every baby is unique, and it may take some time to find the perfect bedtime routine that suits your little one. Be patient, observe your baby's cues, and adjust the routine as needed. By creating a relaxing bedtime routine, you are helping your baby develop healthy sleep habits, which will benefit both of you in the long run.

Natural Remedies for Sleep Difficulties

Sleep difficulties can be a common challenge for both babies and mothers alike. As a mother, it can be distressing to see your little one struggle to fall asleep or wake up frequently during the night. However, there are several natural remedies that can help promote peaceful and restful sleep for your baby. In this subchapter, we will explore these remedies and provide you with practical tips to nurture your baby's sleep patterns naturally.

1. Create a soothing bedtime routine: Establishing a consistent bedtime routine can signal to your baby that it's time to wind down and prepare for sleep. Consider activities such as a warm bath, gentle massage, or reading a calming story. Make sure the environment is dimly lit, quiet, and free from distractions.

2. Use aromatherapy: Essential oils can have a profound impact on sleep quality. Lavender, chamomile, and mandarin are known for their calming properties. Dilute a few drops of these oils in a carrier oil, such as coconut or almond oil, and massage onto your baby's feet or use a diffuser to disperse the scent in the room.

3. Optimize the sleep environment: Ensure your baby's sleep environment is comfortable and conducive to rest. Maintain a cool temperature, use a white noise machine or a fan to drown out any external sounds, and keep the room dark with blackout curtains or a sleep mask.

4. Implement gentle sleep cues: Babies thrive on routine and cues. Incorporate gentle sleep cues, such as a specific blanket or stuffed animal, soft music, or a special bedtime song that you sing before sleep.

5. Herbal remedies: Certain herbs, such as chamomile and passionflower, have calming properties and can aid in promoting sleep. Consult with a naturopathic doctor or pediatrician experienced in herbal medicine to determine the appropriate dosage and preparation for your baby.

6. Breastfeeding for comfort: If your baby wakes up during the night and seems restless, breastfeeding can provide comfort and help them fall back asleep. Breast milk contains natural sleep-inducing hormones that can assist in calming your baby.

Remember, each baby is unique, and what works for one may not work for another. Patience and consistency are key when implementing natural remedies for sleep difficulties. It's important to consult with a naturopathic physician or healthcare professional experienced in baby care to ensure the remedies you choose are safe and appropriate for your little one.

By embracing these natural remedies and nurturing your baby's sleep patterns, you can create a peaceful and restful environment that promotes healthy sleep habits for both you and your little one.

Chapter 6: Building a Strong Immune System

Strengthening the Immune System Naturally

As a mother, your top priority is ensuring the health and well-being of your precious little one. One crucial aspect of baby care is nurturing their immune system, which plays a vital role in protecting them from various illnesses and infections. While conventional medicine has its place, naturopathic methods can also be incredibly effective in strengthening your baby's immune system naturally.

Breastfeeding is a powerful tool in boosting your baby's immunity. Breast milk is rich in antibodies, enzymes, and white blood cells that provide unparalleled protection against pathogens. Aim to breastfeed exclusively for the first six months, and continue breastfeeding alongside solid foods until at least one year of age.

Introducing a diverse range of whole foods is another key factor in bolstering your baby's immune system. Opt for organic produce whenever possible, as it is free from harmful pesticides and chemical residues. Colorful fruits and vegetables are packed with essential vitamins, minerals, and antioxidants that support the immune system. Additionally, include fermented foods like yogurt and sauerkraut to provide beneficial probiotics that promote a healthy gut, where a significant portion of the immune system resides.

Regular physical activity is not only essential for your baby's overall development but also helps strengthen their immune system. Encourage age-appropriate activities that allow them to explore and engage in physical movement. Spending time outdoors exposes your baby to fresh air and natural sunlight, which boosts vitamin D levels, crucial for a robust immune system.

Natural remedies can also provide an extra layer of immune support for your little one. Herbs like echinacea and elderberry have been used for centuries to boost immunity and fight off infections. Consult with a qualified naturopathic practitioner to determine the appropriate dosage and form for your baby.

Lastly, creating a healthy and nurturing environment is paramount. Minimize exposure to toxins by using natural cleaning products, avoiding synthetic fragrances, and opting for organic bedding and clothing. Encourage good hygiene practices, such as frequent handwashing, to prevent the spread of germs.

By following these naturopathic principles, you can help strengthen your baby's immune system naturally and set them on a path towards lifelong health. Remember, each baby is unique, so it's crucial to consult with a healthcare professional experienced in naturopathic baby care to tailor these recommendations to your child's specific needs. Embrace the power of nature and provide your little one with the best possible start in life.

Natural Ways to Prevent and Treat Illnesses

In this subchapter, we will explore the various natural ways to prevent and treat illnesses for your precious baby. As a mother, you understand the importance of ensuring your little one's well-being, and adopting a naturopathic approach to baby care can prove to be highly beneficial.

Prevention is always better than cure, and when it comes to your baby's health, it holds even more significance. One of the most effective ways to prevent illnesses is by breastfeeding. Breast milk contains essential antibodies that boost your baby's immune system, protecting them against various diseases. Additionally, maintaining proper hygiene by regularly washing your hands and ensuring a clean environment for your baby can go a long way in preventing infections.

However, if your baby does fall ill, there are several natural remedies you can try to alleviate their symptoms and support their recovery. For common colds and coughs, steam inhalation with a few drops of eucalyptus or lavender oil can help ease congestion and promote better breathing. You can also create a soothing herbal tea using chamomile or ginger to provide relief from tummy troubles or teething discomfort.

Herbal remedies can be highly effective in treating a range of ailments. For instance, chamomile or lavender oil can be gently massaged onto your baby's skin to calm them and aid in sleep. Alternatively, a warm bath infused with a few drops of chamomile or calendula oil can soothe skin irritations and diaper rashes.

It is important to consult with a naturopathic doctor or a qualified practitioner before trying any natural remedies, as they can guide you on the appropriate dosage or combination of herbs for your baby's specific condition.

In addition to natural remedies, ensuring your baby receives a balanced and nutrient-rich diet is crucial for their overall health. Introducing organic fruits and vegetables and avoiding processed foods can strengthen their immune system and provide essential vitamins and minerals.

Remember, as a mother, you have the power to make informed choices about your baby's health. By adopting a naturopathic approach to baby care, you can protect your little one from illnesses and provide them with the best possible start in life.

Supporting the Immune System through Lifestyle Choices

As a mother, you want nothing more than to ensure the health and well-being of your precious little one. One of the most crucial aspects of your baby's health is their immune system. A strong immune system plays a vital role in protecting your baby from illnesses and infections. In this subchapter, we will explore how you can support your baby's immune system through lifestyle choices, following the principles of naturopathic baby care.

Breastfeeding is a cornerstone of naturopathic baby care, as it provides numerous benefits for your baby's immune system. Breast milk is rich in antibodies, enzymes, and other immune-boosting substances that help protect your baby from infections. Aim to breastfeed exclusively for the first six months and continue breastfeeding alongside the introduction of solid foods to provide ongoing immune support.

Introducing a variety of nutrient-dense foods is another key aspect of supporting your baby's immune system. Focus on whole, organic foods that are free from pesticides, additives, and preservatives. Colorful fruits and vegetables, rich in vitamins, minerals, and antioxidants, help strengthen your baby's immune system. Include probiotic-rich foods like yogurt and fermented vegetables to promote a healthy gut, which plays a crucial role in immune function.

Creating a clean and toxin-free environment for your baby is paramount. Avoid exposing your baby to harsh chemicals found in conventional cleaning products, pesticides, and personal care items. Opt for natural alternatives or consider making your own cleaning products using simple ingredients like vinegar and baking soda. Additionally, ensure your baby's sleeping area is well-ventilated and free from allergens, such as dust mites and pet dander.

Regular exercise and outdoor play are essential for your baby's immune system development. Fresh air, sunlight, and physical activity help stimulate the production of immune-boosting cells and improve overall health. Take your baby for daily walks, play in the park, or engage in gentle activities appropriate for their age.

Lastly, establishing healthy sleep habits is crucial for your baby's immune system. A good night's sleep helps regulate immune function and promotes overall well-being. Create a soothing bedtime routine, provide a comfortable sleep environment, and ensure your baby gets enough restorative sleep each night.

By implementing these lifestyle choices, you can support your baby's immune system naturally and help them grow into a healthy and resilient individual. Remember, every small step you take towards nurturing your baby's immune health today will lay the foundation for a lifetime of well-being.

Chapter 7: Nurturing Emotional Well-being

Encouraging Emotional Bonding

In the early stages of a baby's life, emotional bonding plays a crucial role in their overall development. As a mother, your ability to form a strong emotional connection with your baby is vital in shaping their emotional well-being and fostering a sense of security. By nurturing an emotional bond, you lay the foundation for a healthy and balanced life for your little one. In this subchapter, we will explore various ways to encourage emotional bonding between you and your baby the naturopathic way.

Skin-to-Skin Contact: One of the most effective ways to strengthen the emotional bond with your baby is through skin-to-skin contact. Holding your baby against your bare chest promotes a sense of security, warmth, and comfort. This practice not only regulates your baby's body temperature but also releases oxytocin in both you and your baby, promoting relaxation and bonding.

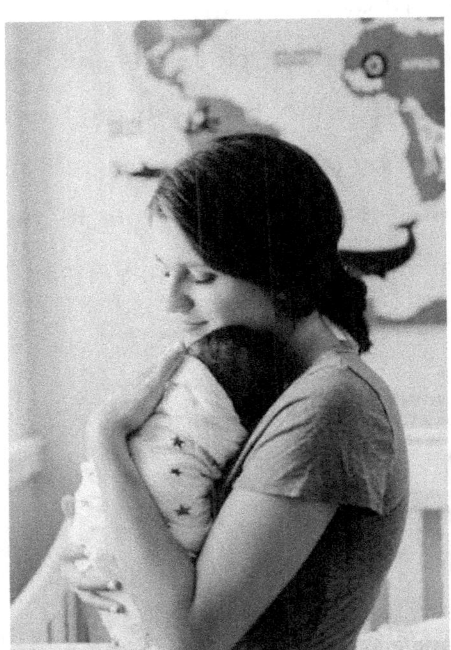

Breastfeeding: Breastfeeding is not only a means of nourishment but also a powerful tool for emotional bonding. The physical closeness, eye contact, and skin-to-skin contact during breastfeeding create a deep emotional connection between mother and baby. It also provides your baby with essential nutrients and antibodies that boost their immune system, promoting overall well-being.

Babywearing: Carrying your baby in a sling or baby carrier keeps them close to your body and allows for constant interaction. Babywearing promotes a strong emotional bond by providing a sense of security, warmth, and familiarity. It also allows you to engage in daily activities while keeping your baby close, ensuring they feel connected to you at all times.

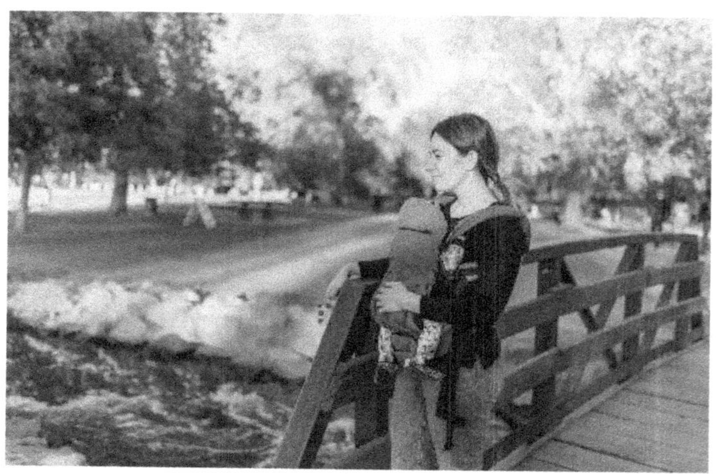

Gentle Touch: Incorporating gentle touch into your daily routine is another effective way to encourage emotional bonding. Massaging your baby using natural oils not only helps in relieving discomforts like colic and constipation but also creates a nurturing and loving environment.

The physical contact and gentle strokes release endorphins, promoting relaxation and enhancing the emotional bond between you and your baby.

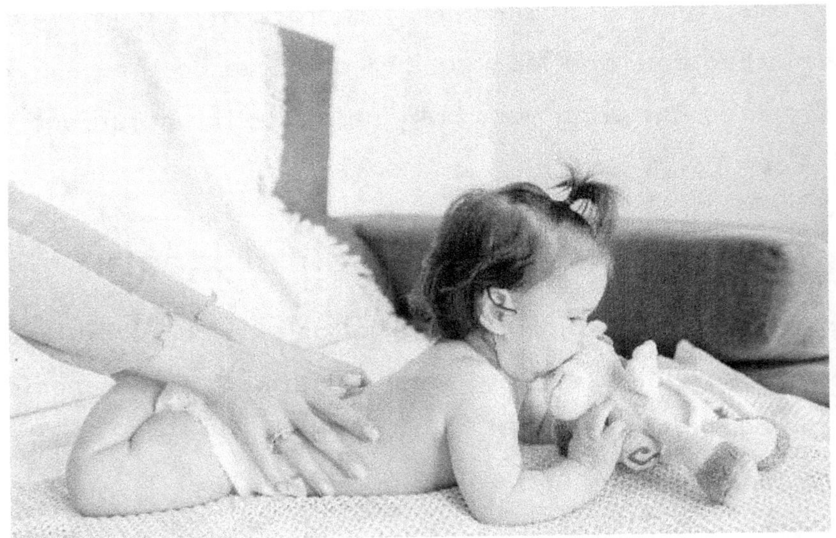

Responsive Parenting: Responding promptly to your baby's needs helps them develop trust and confidence in your care. By understanding and meeting their needs, you create a secure attachment, which is the foundation for healthy emotional development. This entails recognizing and responding to cues, such as hunger, tiredness, or a need for comfort promptly.

By incorporating these naturopathic practices into your baby care routine, you can encourage emotional bonding and create a nurturing environment for your little one. Remember, building a strong emotional bond takes time and patience. Embrace the journey of motherhood, and let your love and care be the guiding force in nurturing your baby naturally, the naturopathic way.

Promoting Positive Mental Health

Mental health is as crucial as physical health, and it is never too early to start nurturing positive mental well-being in your little one. In this subchapter, we will explore various naturopathic approaches to promote positive mental health in babies. By incorporating these practices into your baby care routine, you can provide a solid foundation for their emotional well-being.

1. Bonding and Attachment: The bond between a mother and her baby is the cornerstone of their mental health. Spend quality time with your little one, engaging in activities that encourage eye contact, skin-to-skin contact, and gentle touch. This helps establish a secure attachment, fostering feelings of trust and love.

2. Emotional Expression: Encourage your baby to express their emotions freely. Allow them to cry, laugh, and express joy or frustration without judgment. By acknowledging and validating their emotions, you create a safe space for emotional growth and development.

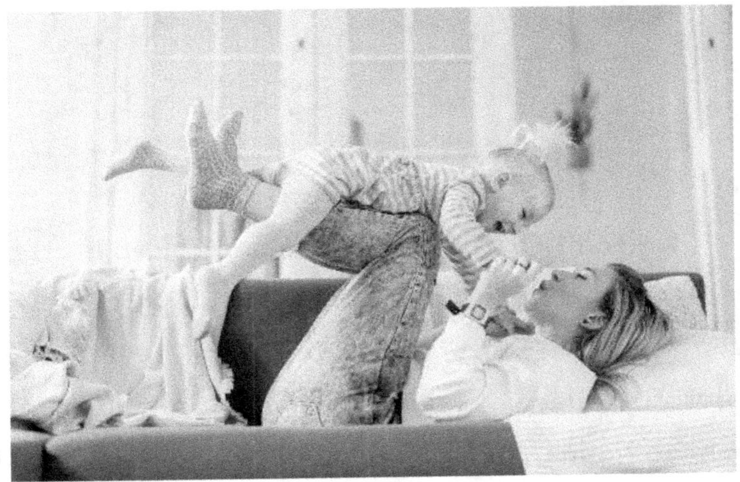

3. Mindful Parenting: Practice mindfulness in your interactions with your baby. Being present in the moment, fully engaged, and attentive to your baby's cues helps create a sense of security and stability, reducing anxiety and promoting positive mental well-being.

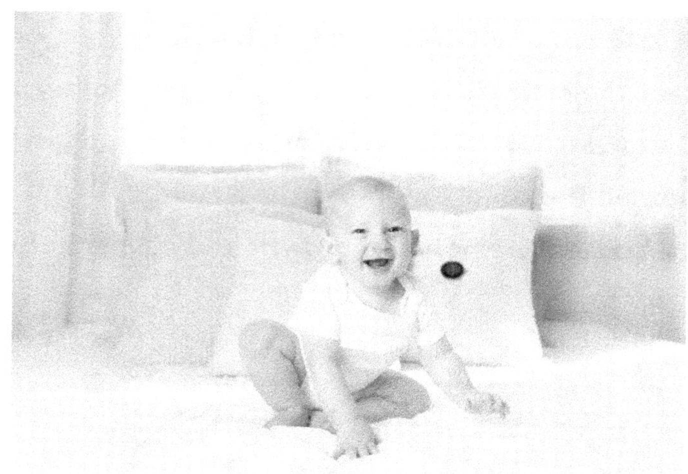

4. Healthy Sleep Habits: Adequate sleep is essential for mental health, even in babies. Establish a consistent sleep routine, ensuring your baby gets enough restorative sleep. Create a calming environment by dimming lights, playing relaxing music, and avoiding stimulating activities before bedtime.

5. Nutritious Diet: A naturopathic approach to baby care emphasizes the importance of a nutrient-rich diet. Provide your baby with a balanced diet that includes fruits, vegetables, whole grains, and lean proteins. Proper nutrition supports brain development, mood regulation, and overall mental well-being.

6. Outdoor Time: Nature has a profound impact on mental health. Take your baby outdoors for a breath of fresh air and exposure to natural surroundings. The sights, sounds, and smells of nature stimulate the senses, promote relaxation, and reduce stress.

7. Limit Screen Time: Excessive screen time can negatively impact mental health, even for babies. Minimize your baby's exposure to screens, including television, smartphones, and tablets. Instead, engage them in interactive play, reading, and social interactions to promote healthy brain development.

Remember, promoting positive mental health is an ongoing process that requires patience, consistency, and love. By incorporating these naturopathic practices into your baby care routine, you can empower your little one with the tools they need for a lifetime of emotional well-being.

Techniques for Soothing and Calming

Babies have unique needs when it comes to soothing and calming techniques. As a mother, it is essential to understand how to provide your little one with natural and nurturing care. In this subchapter, we will explore various techniques for soothing and calming your baby, the naturopathic way.

1. Baby Massage: One of the most effective ways to soothe and bond with your baby is through gentle massage. Using natural oils such as almond or coconut oil, massage your baby's body in soft, rhythmic motions. This technique helps promote relaxation, aids digestion, and improves circulation.

2. Aromatherapy: Harness the power of essential oils to create a calming environment for your baby. Lavender, chamomile, and mandarin are known for their soothing properties. Dilute a few drops of the chosen oil in a carrier oil and diffuse it in the nursery or use it during massage to induce a sense of calmness.

3. Babywearing: Carrying your baby in a sling or carrier not only keeps them close and secure but also provides a soothing environment akin to the womb. The gentle swaying motion and the warmth of your body promote relaxation and reduce fussiness.

4. White Noise: Babies often find comfort in repetitive sounds similar to those they experienced in the womb. Utilize white noise machines or apps that imitate sounds like rainfall, ocean waves, or gentle humming to create a soothing atmosphere for your baby to sleep or relax.

5. Herbal Remedies: Naturopathic remedies, such as herbal teas or infusions, can be used to calm a fussy baby. Chamomile tea, for instance, has mild sedative properties and can help alleviate colic or digestive issues. Consult with a naturopathic practitioner for appropriate herbal remedies suitable for your baby's age and condition.

6. Baby Yoga: Gentle stretches and movements can help calm a restless baby. Baby yoga incorporates simple poses and movements that aid digestion, release tension, and promote relaxation. Joining a baby yoga class or following instructional videos specifically designed for infants can be beneficial.

Remember, every baby is unique, and their response to soothing techniques may differ. Pay attention to your baby's cues and adjust your approach accordingly. By incorporating these natural techniques into your baby's care routine, you can create a calm and nurturing environment that supports their overall well-being.

Disclaimer: It is important to consult with a healthcare professional or a naturopathic practitioner before implementing any new techniques or remedies, particularly if your baby has any pre-existing medical conditions or allergies.

Chapter 8: The Importance of Physical Activity

Developmental Benefits of Physical Activity

Physical activity plays a vital role in a baby's overall development. In this subchapter, we will explore the numerous benefits that physical activity offers to your little one. As a mother, understanding these developmental advantages will empower you to incorporate physical activity into your baby's daily routine, ensuring their optimal growth and well-being.

1. Motor Skills Development: Engaging in physical activities such as crawling, rolling, reaching, and grasping helps your baby develop their gross and fine motor skills. These activities strengthen muscles, improve coordination, and enhance balance, enabling your baby to achieve milestones like sitting, crawling, and eventually walking.

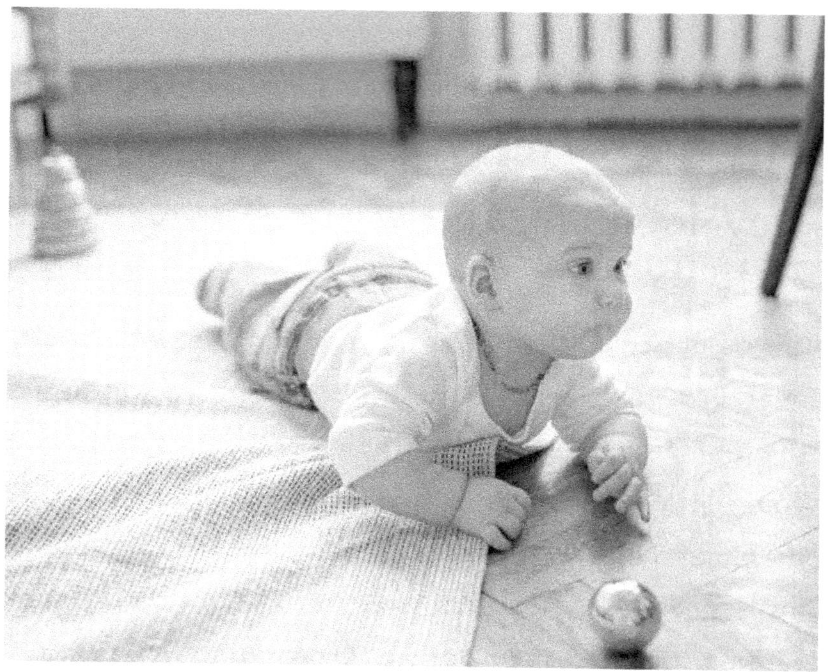

2. Cognitive Development: Physical activity stimulates your baby's brain and promotes cognitive development. As they explore their surroundings, their sensory experiences increase, and they learn to make connections between their actions and the outcomes. This boosts their problem-solving skills, enhances memory, and fosters creativity.

3. Emotional and Social Development: Physical activities involving interaction with others, such as baby yoga classes or playdates, promote social skills and emotional development. These activities encourage bonding, cooperation, and empathy, helping your baby build healthy relationships and develop a sense of self-confidence.

4. Language Development: Engaging in physical activities with your baby provides an excellent opportunity for language development. As you interact

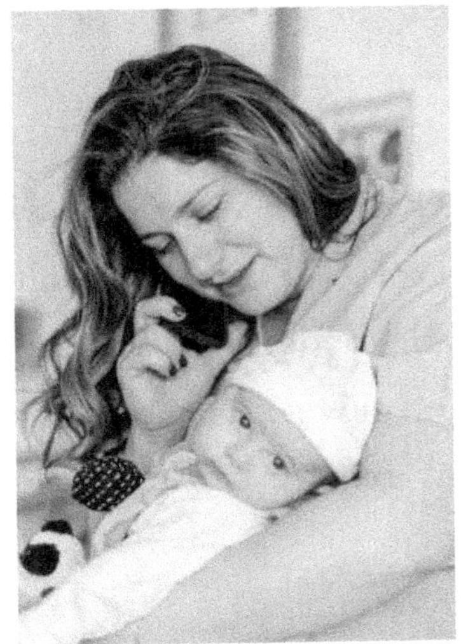

and communicate during these activities, your baby learns new words, gestures, and sounds, expanding their vocabulary and improving their communication skills.

5. Better Sleep Patterns: Regular physical activity helps regulate your baby's sleep patterns and promotes better sleep. Physical exertion during the day allows for deeper and more restful sleep, which is crucial for your baby's growth and development.

6. Enhanced Brain Function: Physical activity increases blood flow to the brain, supplying it with oxygen and essential nutrients. This, in turn, enhances brain function, including memory, attention span, and cognitive abilities.

As a mother embracing the naturopathic approach to baby care, it is important to remember that physical activity should be age-appropriate, safe, and enjoyable for your baby. Consult with your naturopathic doctor or pediatrician to ensure you choose the right activities for your baby's age and developmental stage.

Incorporating physical activity into your baby's routine is not only beneficial for their overall development but also provides a wonderful opportunity for quality bonding time. So, get moving and enjoy the incredible benefits that physical activity offers to your little one's growth and well-being.

Safe and Natural Ways to Encourage Movement

As a mother, you understand the importance of movement for your baby's overall development. Movement not only helps strengthen their muscles and bones but also stimulates their senses and cognitive abilities. In this subchapter, we will explore safe and natural ways to encourage movement for your little one, the naturopathic way.

One of the most effective ways to promote movement is through tummy time. Placing your baby on

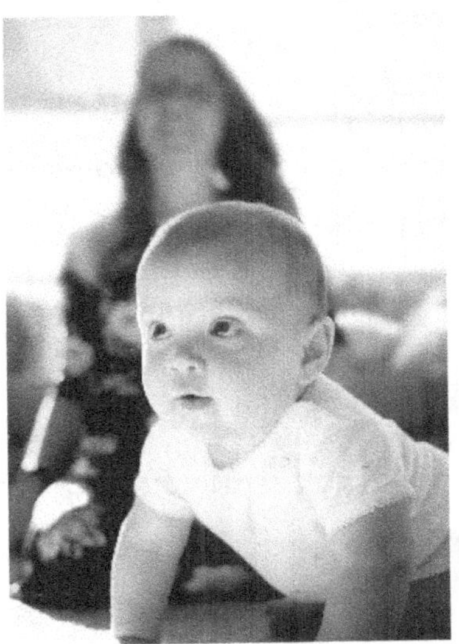

their belly while supervised allows them to engage their neck, shoulder, and back muscles. Start with short sessions and gradually increase the duration as they become more comfortable. You can make this activity more enjoyable by placing colorful toys or a mirror in front of your baby to grab their attention and encourage them to lift their head.

Another natural way to encourage movement is through baby massage. Gentle strokes and kneading not only promote relaxation but also stimulate their muscles and joints. Use a natural oil or cream and make sure to learn the proper techniques from a qualified practitioner or a reliable resource.

Exposing your baby to different textures can also help in their movement development. Place a soft blanket on the floor and encourage them to crawl or roll

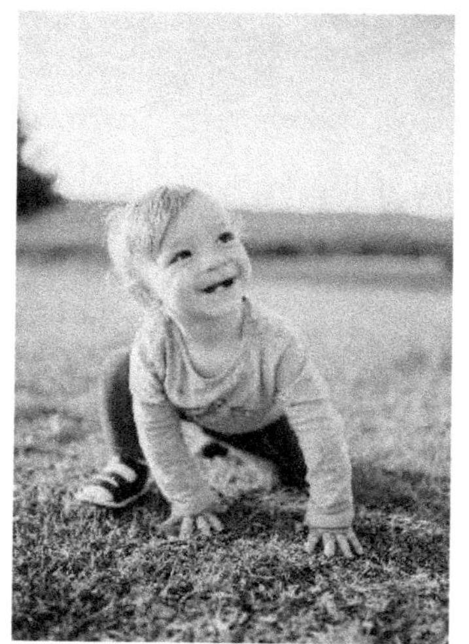

over it. You can also introduce them to varied surfaces like grass, sand, or a textured play mat. These experiences will not only engage their senses but also enhance their coordination and balance.

Incorporating music and rhythm into your baby's routine is another wonderful way to encourage movement. Play soothing tunes or lively songs and gently sway or dance with your baby in your arms. This will not only promote bonding but also stimulate their vestibular system, which is responsible for balance and spatial awareness.

Lastly, avoid confining your baby to restrictive equipment for prolonged periods. While baby carriers, strollers, and bouncers have their place, it is vital to provide ample opportunities for free movement. Allow your baby to explore their surroundings, crawl, and eventually walk at their own pace. Ensure a safe environment by baby-proofing your home and supervising their movements.

By incorporating these safe and natural ways to encourage movement, you are providing your baby with the best foundation for their physical and cognitive development. Embrace the naturopathic approach to baby care and nurture your little one naturally.

Incorporating Nature into Physical Activities

As a mother, you are constantly seeking ways to provide the best care for your little one. One way to promote your baby's overall well-being is by incorporating nature into their physical activities. In this subchapter, we will explore the benefits of connecting with nature and how it can enhance your baby's development.

Nature has a profound impact on human health, and babies are no exception. By exposing your little one to the natural world, you can stimulate their senses, boost their cognitive development, and promote physical growth. Nature offers a wide range of opportunities for physical activities that can be enjoyed by both you and your baby.

Outdoor time is essential for your baby's overall development. It provides them with a diverse sensory experience, helping them to develop their cognitive 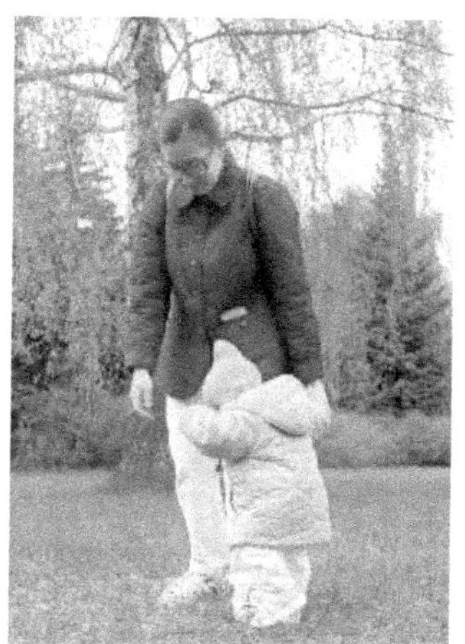 abilities. As you take your baby for a walk in the park, they will be exposed to various textures, sounds, and colors, stimulating their senses and promoting their brain development.

Engaging in physical activities in nature also offers numerous benefits for your baby's physical health. Activities such as hiking, swimming, or even playing in a natural sandbox help to improve their muscle strength, coordination, and balance.

These activities provide an excellent opportunity for your baby to explore their environment, develop their motor skills, and enhance their physical fitness.

Incorporating nature into physical activities also has positive effects on your baby's emotional well-being. Spending time outdoors can reduce stress levels, improve mood, and promote relaxation for both you and your little one. Nature has a calming effect on babies, and the fresh air and natural surroundings can help soothe and relax them.

Additionally, outdoor activities provide an excellent opportunity for you to bond with your baby. Whether it's taking a stroll in the park, playing in the backyard, or going on a nature scavenger hunt, these activities create a special connection between you and your little one. They provide quality time for you to engage with your baby, fostering a strong bond and creating lasting memories.

Incorporating nature into your baby's physical activities is a natural and holistic approach to their overall well-being. By exposing them to the wonders of the natural world, you are providing them with countless benefits for their physical, cognitive, and emotional development. So, go ahead and embrace nature, and watch your baby thrive in its beauty and serenity.

Chapter 9: Naturopathic Baby Care for Special Circumstances

Naturopathic Care for Premature Babies

Premature birth can be a challenging experience for both mother and baby. These tiny miracles require special care and attention to thrive and develop. In this subchapter, we will explore the benefits of naturopathic care for premature babies and how it can support their growth and well-being.

Naturopathic medicine focuses on the body's innate ability to heal itself, using natural remedies and therapies to promote optimal health. When it comes to premature babies, this approach can be particularly effective in supporting their unique needs.

One of the key aspects of naturopathic care for premature babies is nutrition. These tiny infants often have underdeveloped digestive systems, making it crucial to provide them with the right nutrients in a gentle and easily digestible form.

Naturopathic practitioners can guide mothers in choosing the best breast milk or formula options, as well as recommend additional supplements to support the baby's growth and development.

Another important element of naturopathic care is addressing any potential health challenges that premature babies may face. Naturopathic treatments such as herbal medicine, homeopathy, and gentle bodywork can help strengthen their immune system, ease digestive issues, and promote healthy sleep patterns. These natural therapies are safe and gentle, minimizing any potential side effects that conventional medications may have on these delicate infants.

Furthermore, naturopathic care emphasizes the importance of creating a nurturing and supportive environment for premature babies. This includes ensuring they receive adequate sleep, managing their exposure to toxins, and fostering a calm and soothing atmosphere. Naturopathic practitioners can provide guidance on techniques such as baby massage, aromatherapy, and gentle touch to help promote bonding and relaxation.

In addition to the physical well-being of premature babies, naturopathic care also takes into account their emotional and mental development. Mothers are encouraged to engage in activities that promote healthy brain development, such as reading, singing, and interactive play. Naturopathic practitioners can offer suggestions on age-appropriate activities and resources to support the baby's cognitive growth.

In conclusion, naturopathic care offers a holistic and natural approach to supporting the health and well-being of premature babies. By focusing on nutrition, addressing potential health challenges, creating a nurturing environment, and supporting their emotional and mental development, naturopathic medicine can play a vital role in helping these tiny miracles thrive. As a mother, embracing naturopathic care can empower you to provide the best possible care for your premature baby, allowing them to reach their full potential.

Supporting Babies with Allergies Naturally

Allergies can be a challenging issue for both babies and their parents. As a mother, it can be distressing to see your little one suffer from symptoms such as rashes, itching, or digestive disturbances. However, there are natural ways to support and alleviate allergies in babies, without resorting to harsh medications or treatments. In this subchapter, we will explore some effective and gentle methods to nurture your baby with allergies using naturopathic principles.

1. Identify and eliminate triggers: The first step in managing allergies naturally is to identify the specific triggers that may be causing your baby's symptoms. Common culprits include certain foods, environmental allergens, or even products used on their delicate skin. By keeping a journal and monitoring your baby's reactions, you can pinpoint the triggers and eliminate or minimize their exposure.

2. Opt for a nutrient-rich diet: A well-balanced diet plays a crucial role in supporting your baby's immune system and reducing the severity of allergies. Incorporate a variety of fruits, vegetables, whole grains, and lean proteins into their meals. Avoid processed foods, artificial additives, and potential allergens like dairy, wheat, or soy if necessary. Breastfeeding can also provide numerous benefits, as it delivers essential nutrients and immune-boosting properties to your baby.

3. Natural remedies for symptom relief: Naturopathic medicine offers several gentle remedies to alleviate allergy symptoms in babies. For skin issues like rashes or eczema, natural creams or oils containing soothing ingredients like chamomile or calendula can provide relief. A warm bath with colloidal oatmeal or baking soda can also help soothe irritated skin. For respiratory symptoms, a saline nasal spray or steam inhalation can provide temporary relief.

4. Probiotics and gut health: The health of your baby's gut plays a crucial role in their overall immune function. Introducing probiotics, either through breastfeeding or as a supplement, can support a healthy gut flora and reduce the risk of allergies. Consult with a naturopathic practitioner for age-appropriate probiotic recommendations.

5. Avoid unnecessary exposure to toxins: Environmental toxins can exacerbate allergies in babies. Opt for natural and organic household products, detergents, and skincare items. Keep your baby's environment clean and free from dust mites, pet dander, and other potential allergens. Regularly ventilate their sleeping area and use air purifiers if necessary.

Remember, every baby is unique, and what works for one may not work for another. It is crucial to consult with a naturopathic practitioner or pediatrician specializing in natural baby care to develop a personalized plan that meets your baby's specific needs. By taking a holistic and natural approach to supporting your baby with allergies, you can provide them with a nurturing environment and help them thrive.

Naturopathic Approaches to Common Childhood Conditions

As a mother, your baby's health and well-being are of utmost importance to you. The naturopathic approach to baby care offers a gentle and holistic way to address common childhood conditions. By utilizing natural remedies and focusing on preventative measures, you can help your baby thrive and grow in a healthy manner.

One common childhood condition that many babies experience is colic. This can be a distressing time for both you and your little one. Naturopathic approaches suggest gentle techniques such as baby massage, which can help to alleviate discomfort and promote relaxation. Additionally, certain herbal remedies, such as chamomile tea, can be used to soothe the digestive system and reduce colic symptoms.

Another common condition that babies often face is diaper rash. Traditional baby care products can contain harsh chemicals that may further irritate your baby's delicate skin.

Naturopathy recommends using natural remedies such as coconut oil or calendula cream, which have soothing and healing properties. Additionally, allowing your baby's bottom to air dry and using natural fiber diapers can help prevent diaper rash from occurring in the first place.

Ear infections are another common childhood ailment that can cause distress for both babies and parents. Naturopathic approaches focus on boosting the immune system to help prevent such infections. Breastfeeding, if possible, can provide essential antibodies to strengthen your baby's immune system. Additionally, certain herbal remedies, such as echinacea or garlic drops, can be used to support the immune system and reduce the risk of ear infections.

Sleep disturbances can also be a challenge for both babies and parents. Naturopathic approaches suggest establishing a consistent bedtime routine to help your baby relax and prepare for sleep. Additionally, using natural remedies such as lavender essential oil or chamomile tea can promote calmness and improve sleep quality.

By embracing naturopathic approaches to common childhood conditions, you can provide gentle and effective care for your baby. These approaches focus on supporting your baby's natural healing abilities and promoting overall well-being. Remember to consult with a qualified naturopathic practitioner before introducing any new remedies or techniques. Your baby's health is precious, and with naturopathic baby care, you can nurture them naturally.

Chapter 10: Maintaining Balance as a Naturopathic Mother

Self-Care for Mothers

Motherhood is a beautiful and life-altering journey that brings immense joy and fulfillment. However, it can also be overwhelming and exhausting at times. As a mother, it is essential to prioritize your own well-being and practice self-care. By taking care of yourself, you can better care for your little one and create a harmonious environment for both of you. In this subchapter, we will explore self-care practices specifically tailored to mothers, focusing on the naturopathic approach to baby care.

Naturopathic baby care emphasizes the use of natural remedies and holistic approaches to promote the health and well-being of your little one. As a mother, it is crucial to align your self-care practices with this philosophy. Here are some key areas to focus on:

1. Rest and Relaxation: Sleep deprivation is a common challenge for new mothers. Ensure you prioritize rest and aim for quality sleep whenever possible. Take short naps during the day, delegate tasks to others, and create a calm bedtime routine for both you and your baby.

2. Nutrition: A well-balanced diet is vital for your overall health and energy levels. Focus on consuming whole, nutrient-dense foods that provide essential vitamins and minerals. Incorporate plenty of fruits, vegetables, lean proteins, and healthy fats into your meals. Stay hydrated and consider incorporating herbal teas known for their calming and rejuvenating properties.

3. Exercise and Movement: Engaging in gentle exercise and movement can help boost your energy levels, enhance your mood, and relieve stress. Consider activities such as yoga, walking, or postnatal exercises specifically designed for new mothers. Listen to your body and choose activities that feel good and don't strain your recovering body.

4. Emotional Well-being: Motherhood can bring a rollercoaster of emotions. It is crucial to acknowledge and express your feelings. Find healthy outlets for stress, such as journaling, talking to supportive friends or family members, or seeking professional guidance if needed. Practice mindfulness and meditation to cultivate a sense of calm and balance.

5. Time for Yourself: Carve out regular time for yourself, even if it's just a few minutes each day. Engage in activities that bring you joy and recharge your batteries, whether it's reading a book, taking a soothing bath, or pursuing a hobby. Remember, you deserve and need this time to replenish your energy.

By prioritizing self-care, you are not only investing in your own well-being but also creating a positive and nurturing environment for your baby. Remember, you can't pour from an empty cup. So, take care of yourself, mama, because you are the heart and soul of your baby's world.

Balancing Naturopathic Practices with Modern Medicine

In today's world, where modern medicine has made remarkable advancements, it can be challenging for mothers to navigate the world of baby care. As a mother, you want nothing but the best for your little one, and that includes ensuring their health and well-being. This subchapter aims to shed light on the importance of balancing naturopathic practices with modern medicine when it comes to nurturing your baby naturally.

Naturopathic baby care focuses on holistic approaches that emphasize the body's inherent ability to heal itself. It encompasses natural remedies, nutrition, and lifestyle choices that promote overall wellness. While modern medicine is often necessary for acute conditions or emergencies, incorporating naturopathic practices into your baby's routine can complement and enhance their overall health.

One of the key benefits of naturopathic baby care is its emphasis on prevention. By adopting natural remedies and lifestyle choices, you can strengthen your baby's immune system and reduce the risk of illness. Breastfeeding, for instance, is not only a natural way to provide essential nutrients to your baby but also boosts their immune system, protecting them from various infections.

Moreover, naturopathy encourages a focus on nutrition. Introducing wholesome, organic foods to your baby's diet can provide them with vital nutrients, promoting healthy growth and development. This approach also promotes natural remedies such as herbal teas, essential oils, and homeopathy, which can alleviate minor ailments without resorting to synthetic medications.

However, it's essential to strike a balance between naturopathic practices and modern medicine. While naturopathy can provide numerous benefits, there are instances where modern medicine is necessary and even life-saving.

Vaccinations, for instance, play a crucial role in protecting your baby from serious diseases. Consulting with a healthcare professional who embraces both naturopathic and modern medical approaches can help you make informed decisions.

Remember, every baby is unique, and what works for one may not work for another. It's important to be open-minded and flexible when it comes to your baby's healthcare. Finding a healthcare provider who respects your naturopathic beliefs and can work in tandem with modern medicine is essential for achieving optimal results.

In conclusion, the journey of baby care is a delicate balance between naturopathic practices and modern medicine. By embracing naturopathic approaches, you can promote your baby's overall well-being and instill healthy habits from an early age. However, it's crucial to recognize the importance of modern medicine in certain situations. By striking this balance, you can provide your baby with the best of both worlds and ensure their health and happiness.

Creating a Sustainable Lifestyle for the Whole Family

In today's fast-paced world, it is essential for mothers to prioritize creating a sustainable lifestyle for their families. This subchapter aims to guide mothers in embracing a naturopathic approach to baby care while fostering sustainability throughout their daily lives.

Naturopathic baby care emphasizes the use of natural remedies and gentle practices to promote the optimal health and well-being of infants. However, it is equally important to extend this holistic approach beyond just baby care and incorporate sustainable practices that benefit the entire family and the environment.

One of the first steps towards creating a sustainable lifestyle is to prioritize eco-friendly products for your baby. Opt for organic cotton clothing, bedding, and diapers to minimize exposure to harmful chemicals and reduce environmental impact. Additionally, choose natural and non-toxic baby care products, such as organic soaps, shampoos, and lotions, which are not only safe for your baby but also better for the planet.

Another crucial aspect of sustainability is proper waste management. Encourage recycling and composting within your household, teaching your children the importance of reducing waste and conserving resources. Implementing a zero-waste lifestyle can be a rewarding challenge for the entire family, from using reusable cloth diapers and wipes to packing waste-free lunches in reusable containers.

Sustainable nutrition plays a significant role in naturopathic baby care. Introduce your baby to organic, locally sourced, and seasonal foods, promoting a healthy and eco-conscious diet from an early age. Engage in activities like gardening, where you can grow your own herbs and vegetables, teaching your children about the connection between food and the environment.

Energy conservation is another crucial aspect of sustainability. Encourage your family to adopt energy-saving practices such as turning off lights when not in use, using energy-efficient appliances, and reducing water consumption. Teach your children to appreciate and conserve natural resources, emphasizing the importance of preserving the planet for future generations.

By adopting a naturopathic approach to baby care and integrating sustainable practices into your family's lifestyle, you are not only promoting your baby's well-being but also contributing to a healthier and more environmentally conscious future. Embrace the concept of sustainability and make it a way of life for your entire family. Together, we can create a harmonious balance between nature, health, and well-being.

Introducing solid foods to a baby

Introducing solid foods to a baby is an important milestone. When it comes to Indian cuisine for a 1st-year baby, it's crucial to choose nutritious and easily digestible options. Here are 25 vegetarian Indian recipes suitable for babies in their first year:

1. Rice Cereal: Cook rice until soft, mash or blend it with breast milk or formula to a smooth consistency.

2. Khichdi: Combine cooked rice, lentils (moong dal), and vegetables like carrots and peas. Cook until soft and well-mashed.

3. Vegetable Puree: Steam or boil vegetables like carrots, pumpkin, sweet potato, or beetroot, then blend to a smooth puree.

4. Lentil Soup: Cook moong dal or masoor dal with a little turmeric and water until soft, then mash or blend to a soup-like consistency.

5. Potato Mash: Boil and mash potatoes until smooth. Add a little breast milk or formula for a creamy texture.

6. Apple Puree: Steam or boil apples until tender, then blend to a smooth puree. You can add a pinch of cinnamon for flavor.

7. Banana Mash: Mash ripe bananas until smooth and creamy. You can also mix it with breast milk or formula.

8. Spinach Puree: Steam or blanch spinach leaves, then blend to a smooth puree. It can be mixed with rice or lentils.

9. Avocado Mash: Mash ripe avocado until smooth. It's a nutritious option for healthy fats

10.Moong Dal Soup: Cook moong dal with a pinch of turmeric and water. Blend it to a soup-like consistency and add a little ghee for flavor.

11. Carrot and Potato Mash: Steam or boil carrots and potatoes, then mash them together until smooth.

12. Pumpkin Puree: Steam or boil pumpkin cubes until tender, then blend to a smooth puree.

13. Beetroot Puree: Steam or boil beetroot until soft, then blend to a smooth puree. It can be mixed with rice or lentils.

14. Butternut Squash Puree: Steam or boil butternut squash cubes, then blend until smooth. It's packed with vitamins and fiber.

15. Pear Puree: Steam or boil pears until tender, then blend to a smooth puree. It's a great source of dietary fiber.

16. Rice and Lentil Porridge: Cook rice and lentils together until soft and well-mashed. Add water to adjust the consistency.

17. Sweet Potato Mash: Steam or boil sweet potatoes, then mash until smooth. It's a good source of Vitamin A.

18. Papaya Puree: Peel and deseed ripe papaya, then blend to a smooth puree. It aids digestion.

19. Oatmeal Cereal: Cook oats with water until soft and creamy. You can add breast milk or formula for added nutrition.

20. Poha (Flattened Rice) Porridge: Rinse poha, then cook it with water until soft. Add a little ghee for flavor.

21. Pea Puree: Steam or boil green peas until tender, then blend to a smooth puree.

22. Tomato Rice: Cook rice with tomatoes and mild spices until soft and well-cooked. Mash or blend it to an appropriate consistency.

23. Mashed Chickpeas: Boil chickpeas until soft, then mash them until smooth. You can add a little lemon juice for flavor.

24. Cucumber Raita: Grate cucumber and mix it with yogurt. It's a cooling and nutritious option.

25. Cauliflower Mash: Steam or boil cauliflower florets until tender, then mash until smooth. It's a good source of Vitamin C.

Remember to introduce one new food at a time and observe any possible allergic reactions. Consult with your pediatrician before introducing new foods to your baby's diet.

Conclusion: Embracing Naturopathic Baby Care as a Mother

As a mother, the health and well-being of your baby is undoubtedly your top priority. You want to provide them with the best care possible, ensuring their physical, emotional, and mental development. In this journey of motherhood, embracing naturopathic baby care can be a game-changer, offering you a holistic and natural approach to raising a healthy and happy baby.

Naturopathic baby care focuses on supporting your baby's innate healing abilities and promoting optimal health through natural remedies, nutrition, and lifestyle choices. By understanding and implementing these principles, you can create a nurturing environment that sets the foundation for your baby's lifelong wellness.

One of the key aspects of naturopathic baby care is understanding the importance of a natural and balanced diet. Breastfeeding, whenever possible, is highly encouraged as it provides essential nutrients, antibodies, and a strong bond between mother and baby. If breastfeeding is not an option, choosing organic formula without additives and chemicals is the next best choice.

Introducing solid foods to your baby's diet should be done thoughtfully, prioritizing organic, whole foods and avoiding processed or sugary options. Naturopathic principles suggest a gradual introduction of foods, paying attention to any signs of allergies or intolerances. This approach helps to promote healthy digestion and reduce the risk of developing food sensitivities.

Another significant aspect of naturopathic baby care is using natural remedies to address common ailments and promote overall well-being. From diaper rashes and teething discomfort to coughs and colds, there are many effective and safe natural remedies available.

These include herbal teas, essential oils, homeopathic remedies, and gentle massage techniques. By embracing these natural alternatives, you can minimize the use of synthetic medications and their potential side effects.

Additionally, naturopathic baby care emphasizes the importance of creating a nurturing and toxin-free environment. This involves using natural and non-toxic baby products, such as diapers, wipes, and skincare items. It also means minimizing exposure to harmful chemicals found in household cleaning products, plastics, and pesticides.

By embracing naturopathic baby care, you are not only providing your baby with the best start in life, but you are also empowering yourself as a mother. You become an active participant in your baby's health journey, making informed decisions and taking control of their well-being.

As you embark on this naturopathic baby care journey, remember that every baby is unique and may respond differently to various approaches. It is essential to consult with a qualified naturopathic doctor or healthcare professional to tailor the care to your baby's specific needs.

In conclusion, by embracing naturopathic baby care, you are embracing a way of life that prioritizes the natural, holistic, and gentle approach to raising your baby. Your commitment to providing a nurturing and healthy environment will undoubtedly have a profound and lasting impact on your baby's overall well-being. Trust your instincts as a mother, listen to your baby's cues, and embark on this beautiful journey of naturopathic baby care with confidence and love.

Author

Vidyashankar is a Civil engineer by profession who discovered a deep passion for Naturopathy. Alongside his engineering career, he delved into the world of natural healing and wellness, exploring various aspects such as alternative therapies, holistic living, and natural remedies. Driven by his desire to share his knowledge, he began writing books on Naturopathy, offering practical guidance and valuable information for those seeking a balanced and natural approach to health and well-being. With his unique perspective blending scientific principles with the wisdom of natural healing, Vidyashankar presents Naturopathy in a relatable and accessible manner, inspiring readers to embrace a more holistic lifestyle. His dedication to spreading awareness about Naturopathy and his passion for writing have made him a respected author in the field, with his books recognized for their valuable insights, practical tips, and easy-to-understand language. Through his writings, Vidyashankar aims to empower individuals to make informed choices and embark on a journey towards a healthier and harmonious life.

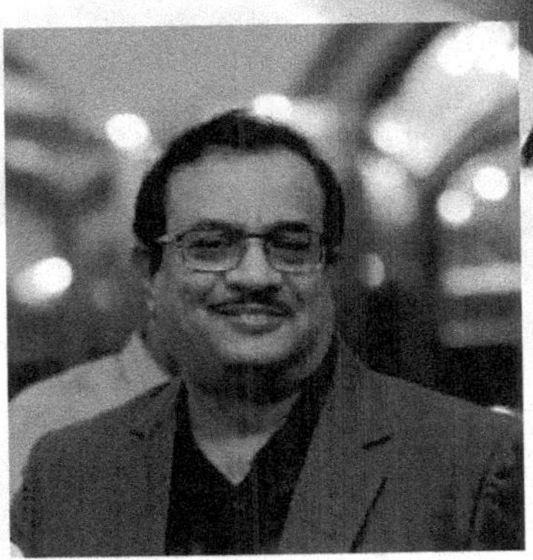